POCKET
Vitan

ANTI-AGEING ANTIOXIDANT

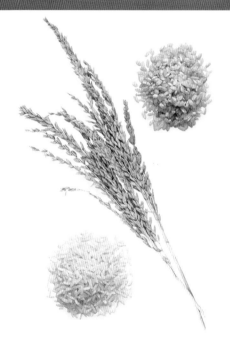

Stephanie Pedersen

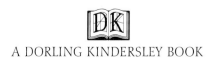

A DORLING KINDERSLEY BOOK

CONTENTS

VITAMIN BASICS

The word "vitamin" is a relatively new term. The word first appeared in dictionaries in 1912 and was coined to describe the organic substances in food essential for most chemical processes in the body. Before vitamins were discovered, doctors recommended food itself: carrots (rich in vitamin A) to maintain vision, citrus fruit (high in vitamin C) to prevent scurvy, and whole grains and legumes (abundant in vitamin B1) to ward off beriberi.

Scientists have identified 13 vitamins that are considered essential for health – essential because the body does not manufacture these nutrients itself. In other words, these vitamins must come either from food or from supplements. Essential vitamins are grouped into two categories: fat-soluble and water-soluble.

Essential fat-soluble vitamins include vitamins A, D, E, and K. These are stored in the body's fat to be used as needed. Because the body stockpiles fat-soluble vitamins, it is possible to take too much of one or more of these vitamins, although this rarely occurs. Vitamin overdose can lead to various symptoms, including headaches and irritability.

The essential water-soluble vitamins are C, B1, B2, B3, B5, B6, B12, folic acid, and biotin. These are not stored in the body: the body uses just what it needs at any given time and excretes the unused amount in the urine.

Two important points about vitamins. Many people believe that if they take nutritional supplements, they won't have to worry about a balanced diet. But vitamins are just that, supplements. It is important to remember that the human body is designed to absorb vitamins from food. In addition, science is rapidly discovering dozens of health-supportive phytonutrients in food that work with vitamins to promote health and these phytonutrients are unavailable in pill form.

Another important point to remember when it comes to vitamins is that you can have too much of a good thing. While large amounts of some vitamins are helpful in specific situations, too much may cause side effects that range from the merely annoying (such as dry skin or sleep disturbances) to the truly dangerous (such as liver damage).

· HOW TO TAKE · VITAMIN SUPPLEMENTS

◆ Take vitamin supplements with food to increase absorption. Fat-soluble vitamins should be eaten with food containing some fat.

◆ If you experience nausea within a half-hour after taking a vitamin, you may not have had enough food in your stomach.

◆ High doses of vitamins should not be taken at one time. For most efficient absorption, space dosages throughout the day.

WHAT IS VITAMIN E?

Vitamin E is one of the most popular supplements. And with good reason. It is a powerful, fat-soluble antioxidant, responsible for protecting the fatty parts of the body's cells from attack by free radicals. In excess – from sources such as cigarette smoke, air pollutants, or UV light, for example – free radicals can cause damage to cells that may eventually lead to diseases such as heart disease and cancer. Vitamin E also protects the heart by preventing cholesterol from assuming its "oxidized" or artery-clogging form. Additionally, the vitamin is needed to protect red blood cells and for the repair and renewal of tissues – hence its role in wound healing, muscle conditions, and joint diseases.

Despite its wide-ranging importance, vitamin E is a recent discovery. It was first identified in 1922 when researchers found that rats fed a limited diet became infertile. However, after receiving wheat germ oil – which happens to be high in vitamin E – the rats became fertile again. When the responsible nutrient was isolated, scientists named it tocopherol, after the Greek words *tokos* and *phero*, which mean "offspring" and "to bear".

Vitamin E is a fat-soluble vitamin that is actually comprised of two families of compounds: the tocopherols (alpha, beta, gamma, and delta) and the tocotrienols (alpha, beta, gamma, and delta). Of all its constituents, alpha-tocopherol, delta-tocopherol, and gamma-tocopherol are the most studied–although all vitamin E constituents are beneficial.

Unlike the other fat-soluble vitamins – A, D, and K – vitamin E is not effectively stored in the body. After ingestion, it finds its way to the intestines, where it is absorbed along with fat and bile salts into the lymphatic system and then into the blood, which carries it to the liver to be used or stored. Over half of any excess may be lost in the faeces, but some vitamin E is stored in the fatty tissues and the liver, and to a lesser degree, in the heart, muscles, testes, uterus, adrenal and pituitary glands, and blood. Vitamin E is also partially absorbed through the skin when used as an ointment or oil application.

Vitamin E is found in small amounts in animal foods. Yet it is plant foods that are richest in the vitamin. In fact, the best sources of vitamin E are cold-pressed oils from nuts, seeds, and vegetables. Unfortunately, during the modern refinement and purification of oils, grains, flours, fruits, and vegetables, vitamin E is lost. Interestingly, the byproducts of today's refining processes, which are rich in vitamin E, are used to make vitamin E supplements. Based on what we know about vitamin E and its action in the body, many experts feel that an intake of 75–800mg daily is safe and effective. By comparison the EU Recommended Daily Allowance is just 10mg. For that reason, throughout the book, a range of vitamin E dosages are offered.

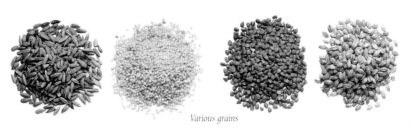

Various grains

FOOD SOURCES

Food is an important, easily digested source of a wide range of vitamins. The following foods are particularly rich in vitamin E:

- Almonds
- Avocados
- Brown rice
- Cold-pressed nut and vegetable oils
- Desiccated liver
- Dried beans
- Leafy greens
- Hazelnuts
- Kelp
- Oatmeal
- Organ meats
- Peanut butter
- Soybeans
- Sweet potatoes
- Sunflower seeds
- Walnuts
- Wheatgerm
- Wholewheat flour

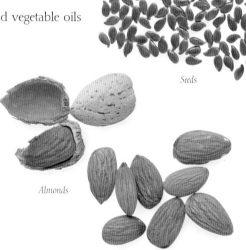

Seeds

Almonds

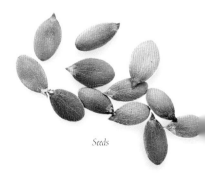

Seeds

NATURAL OR SYNTHETIC?

What kind of vitamin E is best for you – natural or synthetic? It seems that the natural variety is better absorbed in the body. In one study, researchers gave healthy, hospitalized, and seriously ill patients equal doses of natural and synthetic vitamin E together. Blood levels of natural vitamin E were consistently twice those of synthetic, and the same pattern of retention occurred in various organs and glands. Labels indicate natural vitamin E as "d-alpha-tocopherol"; synthetic vitamin E is listed as "dl-alpha-tocopherol".

· HOW MUCH DO I TAKE? ·

How many times have you stood in front of the vitamin shelves in your local health food store or pharmacy and compared labels? And how many times have you wondered why one brand offers 60mg of vitamin C when another boasts 1000mg of vitamin C? Or why another product has 180mcg of folate when a competing brand features 400mcg of the same nutrient? And perhaps more importantly, which one is better? Basic requirements can be satisfied by taking the Recommended Daily Allowance (RDA) needed to avoid nutritional deficiency diseases such as beriberi, rickets, or scurvy. However, many researchers, medical experts, and health authorities believe that the body needs much higher levels of vitamins for optimum health. And in the presence of illness, pollution, prescription medication, or stress, the body may need still higher levels. For this reason, throughout this book, we suggest a range of vitamin dosages. In most cases there are only averages and a little more or a little less may work equally well. If you want to find out the best level to suit you, consult a qualified nutritionist.

SPECIAL NEEDS

While a daily dose of 12 to 15 IU of vitamin E is recommended, the following individuals have increased needs for vitamin E:

SMOKERS Smoking increases the production of free radicals. Levels of vitamin E can become depleted as the vitamin zaps excess free radicals.

ALCOHOLICS Alcohol increases the need for vitamin E.

INDIVIDUALS WHO EAT ONLY COOKED FRUITS OR PROCESSED FRUITS AND VEGETABLES Canning, cooking, and freezing break down the vitamin E in foods.

INDIVIDUALS WHO LIVE IN POLLUTED ENVIRONMENTS OR WHO ARE EXPOSED TO SECONDHAND SMOKE Pollution and secondhand smoke stress the immune system, thus depleting vitamin E levels in the body.

THE ELDERLY With age comes a reduced ability to absorb vitamin E.

INDIVIDUALS WHO EAT FRIED AND DEEP-FRIED FOODS DAILY When oils are heated to a certain temperature they become oxidized, which can stimulate the formation of free radicals in the body. Free radicals are believed to contribute to cancer and vitamin E helps to neutralize them.

VITAMIN E DEFICIENCY

True vitamin E deficiency is very rarely observed in the general population. Any damage caused by deficiency would occur at a cellular, sub-clinical level and symptoms could take years to show themselves. However, there is clinical evidence of vitamin E deficiency occurring in individuals with chronic malabsorption syndromes as well as in premature infants. The value of boosting intake of antioxidants such as vitamin E has more to do with promoting optimal health than combating symptoms of deficiency.

· TOO MUCH OF A GOOD THING ·

Although it is fat-soluble, vitamin E is considered non-toxic because it is not harmful except in extremely high doses. Most experts agree that the upper safe level for daily consumption over a long period is 800mg. In the US leading scientists have recently recommended the upper level could be set at 1000mg daily, since no adverse effects should be expected up to this level.

Oral intake of vitamin E slows blood coagulation somewhat. Therefore it can intensify an existing coagulation defect produced by vitamin K deficiency (vitamin K deficiency can result from either malabsorption or anticoagulant therapy). Supplemental vitamin E may be contraindicated in such conditions.

However, vitamin E has not been found to produce coagulant problems in individuals who are not vitamin K deficient. As with all supplements, patients on medications or under a doctor's care for medical conditions should consult with their practitioner before starting a supplement.

HERBAL LABELLING

You may have wondered why many herbal remedies don't give a clear indication of their potential use on the label. For example, you may be taking ginkgo to boost your memory, dong quai to help regulate your hormones, or St John's wort to lift depression but the packaging won't tell you that this is what the herb does. The reason is that only a proportion of herbs on the market are medically licensed: these are allowed to indicate their therapeutic uses but others, classified as normal foods, can't.

If a licensed formulation is available you may want to choose it instead of an unlicensed one because you can be sure that it contains efficacious ingredients and is made to the highest possible pharmaceutical standards.

UNLICENSED HERBS

Unlicensed herbal remedies are not necessarily any lower in quality. Most are made to the same reputable standards as licensed herbal formulations, and because they are technically "foods" they have to comply with strict food safety rules so that they do not harm human health. Getting a medical licence can take years, so it is no wonder that manufacturers produce herbal supplements without a licence to the highest possible standards.

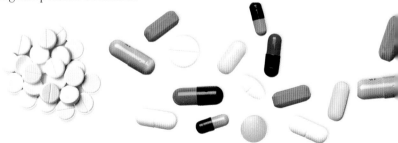

· MAKING THE BEST SELECTION ·

Whichever herbal supplement you choose, here are some guidelines:

◆ Choose a reputable manufacturer whose name you trust, or get advice from a herbalist or health professional.

◆ With tablets and capsules, compare dosages carefully. Some manufacturers may mislead by claiming a powdered herb is an extract, for example (an extract can be as much as 50 times stronger), or standardize herbs to a lower activity than other, more expensive, makes.

◆ Only choose herbal remedies that are properly sealed in tamper-resistant packaging and which have been clearly marked with a "best before" date. Check there is a contact address in case of any problem with the product.

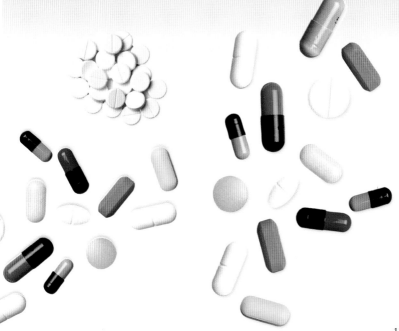

ALZHEIMER'S DISEASE

SYMPTOMS Alzheimer's can strike people in their 40s or 50s and older. In fact, about every one in ten people over the age of 65 is diagnosed with Alzheimer's and millions have the disease worldwide.

Alzheimer's is an incurable disease that destroys brain cells, usually those of the cerebral cortex—causing dementia. Symptoms appear progressively, usually in this order: forgetfulness, shortening of attention span, disintegration of personality, disorientation, memory loss, confusion, restlessness, inability to read, wandering, lack of patience, loss of impulse control, inappropriate behaviour, aggressiveness, irritability, cursing, uncoordination, delusions, hallucinations, loss of language, lack of bladder and bowel control, and inability to feed oneself.

Currently, there is no diagnostic test for Alzheimer's; the most foolproof test for the disease is an autopsy to examine brain tissue. That said, doctors can make an accurate diagnosis in up to 90 per cent of all cases after a careful medical history and physical examination. It's not known exactly what causes Alzheimer's. Some researchers believe it is an inflammatory response to infection; others blame it on free radicals, environmental toxins, or lack of blood flow to the brain. Whatever the culprit, genetics is often a factor.

HOW VITAMIN E CAN HELP Right now there is no cure for Alzheimer's disease. However, vitamin E has been shown by several studies to be an effective companion therapy to other herbal and nutritional treatments in delaying the onset of the disease or lessening its severity. Vitamin E is an antioxidant that helps prevent brain cells from free radical damage. It is also an anticoagulant that thins thickened blood, making it easier for red blood cells to reach the brain. Furthermore, autopsies show that Alzheimer's victims are found to have radically reduced levels of vitamin E in their bodies.

DOSAGES Take up to 800–1000mg of vitamin E daily with meals. In addition, consume daily servings of foods rich in vitamin E, such as avocados, brown rice, dark green leafy vegetables, nuts, oatmeal, seeds, soybeans, and wheatgerm.

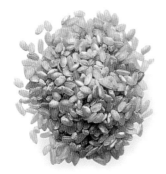

Brown rice

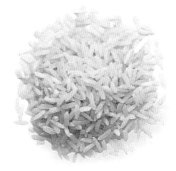

White rice

PRE-ECLAMPSIA

SYMPTOMS Pre-eclampsia is a condition in which blood pressure rises dangerously during pregnancy, putting both the health of the baby and mother at risk. It occurs in about 10-15 per cent of women having their first child, and each year in the UK about 10 mothers and 1000 babies die from its effects.

Many women with pre-eclampsia have no symptoms, which makes attending ante-natal checks extremely important. Throughout the pregnancy, and especially after 20 weeks, the doctor or midwife will check for undesirable rises in blood pressure, and also for the presence of protein in the urine – signs that the condition may be developing.

Fortunately there have been major increases in the understanding of pre-eclampsia in recent years, and it is now thought that dietary factors, especially antioxidant nutrients such as vitamin E, may play an important role in preventing the disease.

HOW VITAMIN E CAN HELP Most researchers agree that an important contributory factor in the development of pre-eclampsia is the action of free radicals – highly reactive and destructive by-products of metabolism that can "oxidize" or damage our cells and tissues. When women consume more vitamin E they may be helping to protect themselves because the nutrient mops up the free radicals that cause the problem.

DOSAGES With medical advice, take 100-400mg daily with meals. In addition, consume daily servings of foods rich in vitamin E as avocados, brown rice, dark green leafy vegetables, nuts, oatmeal, seeds, soybeans, and wheatgerm.

· PRE-ECLAMPSIA RESEARCH ·

A study carried out in the UK in 1999 reported a 76 per cent lower risk of developing pre-eclampsia for women taking 1000mg vitamin C and 268mg natural vitamin E daily compared with placebo capsules. Women at genetic risk or who had suffered from pre-eclampsia in a previous pregnancy were included in the study, taking the vitamins every day between the 16th and 22nd weeks of pregnancy. Because the results showed such a success in high-risk women, trials are now warranted to show whether vitamin supplementation can affect the occurance of pre-eclampsia in women at lower risk.

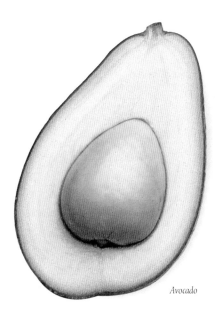

Avocado

ASTHMA

SYMPTOMS Asthma is an inflammation of the airways caused by an allergic reaction. Although not all sufferers are allergic to the same substances, some common triggers are animal hairs, dust mites, mould spores, and pollen. When a trigger is inhaled, the body's antibodies react with the allergen, producing allergen-suppressing histamine and other chemicals. Also, chest muscles constrict, the bronchial lining swells, and the body creates more mucus, thus causing breathing difficulties, coughing (sometimes accompanied by mucus), painless tightness in the chest, and wheezing.

HOW VITAMIN E CAN HELP While vitamin E cannot cure asthma, it has been shown to protect cells in the delicate lining of the lungs. How does it work? Vitamin E is an antioxidant. This is important because asthma attacks frequently occur when the lungs are under stress from allergens. These allergens produce free radicals that weaken the smooth muscle wall of the bronchi. Vitamin E can help quench the oxidants, preventing them from weakening the lungs and provoking an asthma attack.

DOSAGES Take up to 800mg of vitamin E daily with meals. In addition, consume daily servings of foods rich in vitamin E as avocados, brown rice, dark green leafy vegetables, nuts, oatmeal, seeds, soybeans, and wheatgerm.

· ASTHMA SUFFERERS ·

If you suffer from asthma, you're not alone. In Britain there are more than three million sufferers, including one in seven school children, and one in 25 adults. American statistics indicate a 78.6 per cent increase in asthma among under-18s since 1982.

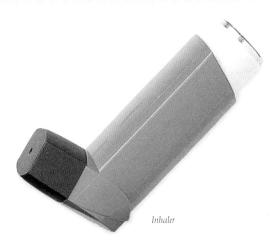

Inhaler

CANCER

SYMPTOMS Cancer occurs when cells begin growing abnormally, forming malignant tumours. These malignant tumours can appear in the breast, the bones, the throat, the brain, the stomach – actually, in almost any area of the body. But why do cells begin acting strangely in the first place? It's believed that exposure to carcinogens causes free radical damage to the cells, which in turn prompts cells to mutate. Common carcinogens include cigarette smoke, fatty foods, industrial chemicals, insecticides, nuclear radiation, pesticides used on food, polluted air, and UV (ultraviolet) light. While cancer symptoms vary widely depending on what part of the body is affected, general signs include blood in the urine or stool, fatigue, hoarseness, indigestion, nagging cough, sores that do not heal, thickening somewhere in the body, and unexplained weight loss.

HOW VITAMIN E CAN HELP While vitamin E cannot wipe out established cancers, it is a powerful antioxidant. In other words, it has the power to stop free radical damage at a cellular level. Several epidemiological studies have shown that individuals who eat large amounts of foods rich in vitamin E each day have significantly lower cancer rates than individuals who eat foods containing little or no vitamin E.

DOSAGES To keep up body levels of protective vitamins E, take 100–400mg of vitamin E daily with meals. In addition, consume daily servings of foods rich in vitamin E, such as avocados, brown rice, dark green leafy vegetables, nuts, oatmeal, seeds, soybeans, and wheatgerm.

· CANCER FACTS ·

◆ There are more than 100 different varieties of cancer.

◆ People with breast cancer have been found to have lower-than-normal levels of vitamin E and the mineral selenium—two important antioxidants that neutralize free radicals.

◆ African-Americans have the highest incidence of prostate cancer, while Asian-Americans have the lowest.

◆ It is believed that intestinal cancer takes up to 20 years to develop.

◆ The single most avoidable cancer risk is smoking.

◆ People whose mothers smoked during pregnancy are about 50 per cent more likely than children of nonsmoking mothers to develop cancer later in life.

CORONARY ARTERY DISEASE

SYMPTOMS Coronary artery disease accounts for about one in three deaths worldwide each year. The disease progresses slowly over the course of years and even decades, but its impact can be instantaneous: In nearly one-third of all cases, death occurs without any previous warning of disease. Indeed, some people have no symptoms, while others may experience chest pain, constriction or a sense of heaviness in the chest, fatigue, pallor, shortness of breath, swelling in the ankles, and weakness. Coronary artery disease occurs when cholesterol deposits build up on coronary artery walls. These special blood vessels provide oxygen and nutrients to the muscles of the heart. When they are unable to deliver adequate blood flow, however, the heart muscle begins to weaken, leading to angina (chest pain), congestive heart failure, and heart attack. When it comes to causes, a high-fat diet is most often implicated, although heredity, stress, inactivity, smoking, and alcoholism are also culprits.

HOW VITAMIN E CAN HELP Vitamin E helps prevent cholesterol from undergoing oxidation, which can increase its chances of being deposited in artery walls, so helping to keep the blood flowing freely around the body.

DOSAGES Take 1400–800mg of vitamin E daily with meals. In addition, consume daily servings of foods rich in vitamin E, such as avocados, brown rice, dark green leafy vegetables, nuts, oatmeal, seeds, soybeans, and wheatgerm.

Note: *Don't take vitamin E without medical advice if you are on anticoagulant therapy.*

· HOW MUCH VITAMIN E IS ENOUGH? ·

While the EU RDA for vitamin E is just 10mg, many experts feel it should be much higher. Researchers point to studies such as a recent double-blind, placebo-controlled intervention trial that showed a significant decrease in nonfatal heart attacks in high-risk subjects (individuals with high cholesterol and/or high blood pressure, smokers, and subjects with a history of heart attacks) who consumed either 268mg or 536mg of vitamin E supplements per day. In comparison, a Finnish clinical trial did not observe any benefit against heart disease when vitamin E was given at a more modest daily dose of 33mg to long-term heavy smokers.

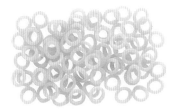
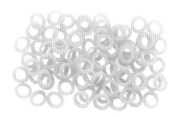

Pasta

HIGH BLOOD CHOLESTEROL

SYMPTOMS Cholesterol is a type of "sticky" substance that can be raised in the blood through eating high levels of saturated fats (found especially in animal foods). Cholesterol thickens blood and gets stuck on artery walls, thus increasing one's risk of coronary artery disease, heart attack, and stroke. Symptoms can include chest pain, lethargy, pallor, and shortness of breath. However, the condition is often asymptomatic; many individuals learn they have high cholesterol only after a routine blood test.

HOW VITAMIN E CAN HELP Vitamin E does not lower cholesterol but it can help to prevent cholesterol from becoming oxidized. Oxidation of cholesterol is what changes it into its particularly dangerous form.

DOSAGES Take 800mg of vitamin E daily with meals. In addition, consume daily servings of foods rich in vitamin E, such as avocados, brown rice, dark green leafy vegetables, nuts, oatmeal, seeds, soybeans, and wheatgerm.

· HEALTH BENEFITS ·

Researchers in the US found that individuals who ate more than 130g (5oz) of nuts rich in vitamin E per week had one-third fewer heart attacks than those who rarely or never ate nuts. Preliminary results from a companion study, indicate that eating nuts may provide the same health benefits to men. Another study of 40,000 postmenopausal women found that those who ate the most nuts reduced their risk of coronary artery disease by 60 per cent.

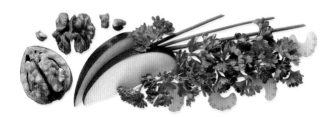

POOR IMMUNITY

SYMPTOMS Reduced immunity can show itself in the form of increased susceptibility to colds, influenza, and mild infections. It can also increase the risk of more serious diseases including cancer. Two main causes of poor immunity are poor diet and stress.

HOW VITAMIN E CAN HELP Vitamin E helps to neutralise free radicals, which in excess can weaken the immune system. There is good data suggesting that vitamin E can also correct the age-related decline in immune function that predisposes older people to infections. In one study in the US, 536mg of vitamin E was given to healthy people aged 60-80 years old. There was significant improvement in the delayed type hypersensitivity skin test – a measure of the vigour of the immune response. In addition, there was an increased ability of the white blood cells to respond to challenges and a very significant increase in interleukin 2 – a growth factor for immune cells. Moreover, vitamin E reduced the production of PGE2 – a substance that is an inhibitor of immune response.

DOSAGES To help improve immune response take 400–800mg of vitamin E daily with meals. In addition, consume daily servings of foods rich in vitamin E, such as avocados, brown rice, dark green leafy vegetables, nuts, oatmeal, seeds, soybeans, and wheatgerm.

Note: *If you are currently on anticoagulant medication, consult with a doctor before taking more than 100 mg of vitamin E daily.*

· CAN YOU GET ENOUGH · VITAMIN E FROM FOOD?

The average daily intake of vitamin E is under 20mg and even the healthiest diet is unlikely to provide more than 30mg. To get 100mg of vitamin E – the minimal amount that may be optimal – you would have to eat the following:

◆ 1389 slices (50kg) wholemeal bread (107,500 kcal)

◆ 833 bowls (25kg) cornflakes (90,000 kcal)

◆ 182 (9.1kg) boiled eggs (13,230 kcal)

◆ 5.8kg boiled spinach (1,102 kcal)

◆ 15.2kg roasted, salted peanuts (91,500 kcal)

◆ 2.1 litres olive oil (17,620 kcal)

CERVICAL DYSPLASIA

SYMPTOMS Cervical dysplasia is an asymptomatic condition found most often in women between the ages of 25 and 35. It has been linked to sexually transmitted diseases, such as the human papillomavirus (HPV), which causes genital warts. Infection by sexually transmitted organisms may be accompanied by oxidants, which can damage cervical cell DNA. Eventually, this cellular damage can lead to cancer.

HOW VITAMIN E CAN HELP Recent research has found that vitamin E can prevent cervical cells from becoming precancerous. The vitamin is a powerful antioxidant, which prevents infected cervical cells from being attacked by cancer-causing oxidants.

DOSAGES Take 100-400mg of vitamin E daily with meals. In addition, consume daily servings of foods rich in vitamin E, such as avocados, brown rice, dark green leafy vegetables, nuts, oatmeal, seeds, soybeans, and wheatgerm.

· CERVICAL DYSPLASIA AND VITAMIN E ·

Researchers at the Lublin Medical Academy in Poland evaluated 168 female patients with normal smears who had not been infected by the human papillomavirus and compared the results to 228 patients with cervical dysplasia who were infected with the human papillomavirus. Members of the second group showed significantly lower levels of vitamin E in their blood than members of the first group.

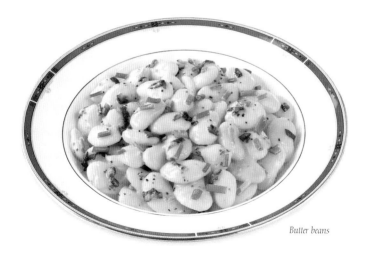

Butter beans

OESTROGEN FACTS

◆ Some 10 million women in the US – about one-fourth of those at or past menopause – regularly take artificial oestrogen (the female sex hormone) supplements, with or without additional supplements of progesterone (the other female sex hormone).

◆ It is believed that one-fifth of women who are prescribed oestrogen never fill their prescription.

◆ A recent survey has found that one-third of women prescribed oestrogen stop taking it within nine months, and more than half stop within a year.

◆ Women's bones slowly begin to lose minerals and become less dense even before menopause. Oestrogen supplements have been proven to reduce the bone loss associated with osteoporosis. Unless a woman is taking oestrogen, she has about a one-in-four chance of developing serious osteoporosis.

◆ Various studies have suggested that oestrogen use increases a woman's risk of breast cancer by as much as 30 per cent.

◆ Statistics show that women who take oestrogen are 40 per cent less likely to develop Alzheimer's disease than individuals who don't take the hormone. Furthermore, the longer an individual takes oestrogen, the more their risk is reduced.

◆ Oestrogen replacement seems to help prevent heart disease in older women. Without oestrogen replacement, a woman's risk of heart attack becomes equal to a man's within 15 years of the menopause.

◆ A report from a 10-year study of 48,470 nurses – one of the largest studies to date – found that oestrogen use reduced the risk of major coronary disease and fatal cardiovascular disease by half.

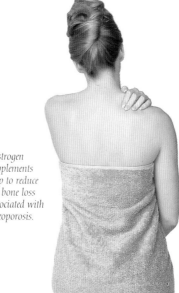

Oestrogen supplements help to reduce the bone loss associated with osteoporosis.

FIBROCYSTIC DISEASE

SYMPTOMS Benign breast disease, chronic cystic mastitis, lumpy breasts, and mammary dysplasia are all names for fibrocystic disease, a condition characterized by one or more lumps in one or both breasts. These lumps may or may not be painful and may be accompanied by greenish or straw-coloured discharge from the nipples. Unlike malignant tumours, these benign lumps are actually cysts, fluid-filled sacs that tend to get bigger toward the end of the menstrual cycle, when the body retains more fluid. Some cysts can be tiny, others can be the size of an egg. It isn't known exactly what causes fibrocystic disease, although an imbalance of ovarian hormones is believed to play a role. The disease occurs mainly in women between the ages of 25 and 50 and usually disappears with menopause.

HOW VITAMIN E CAN HELP Several studies have shown that vitamin E is useful in shrinking or eliminating the cysts associated with fibrocystic disease. It is not known how vitamin E can do this but an indirect effect on hormone regulation is one possibility.

DOSAGE Take 100-400mg of vitamin E daily with meals. In addition, consume daily servings of foods rich in vitamin E, such as avocados, brown rice, dark green leafy vegetables, nuts, oatmeal, seeds, soybeans, and wheatgerm.

· LIMIT CHEMICAL EXPOSURE ·

It's nearly impossible to avoid all chemical toxins in today's world. There is ammonia in cleaning products, chlorine in the water, lead in old paint and pipes, dibromochloropropane in pesticides, carbon monoxide from auto exhaust, and toluene, trichloroethylene, and formaldehyde from printers, photocopiers, and fax machines. Many of these toxins have been linked to allergies, breathing problems, cancer, headaches, infertility, lethargy, lung conditions, reduced attention span, and violence. Ideas for lessening toxins include using environmentally sound dry cleaning, drinking filtered water, purchasing (or making) environmentally-friendly cleaning products, limiting the amount of driving you do, and adding a few chemical-filtering plants such as dracaena, chrysanthemum, and weeping fig (ficus) to your home.

MENOPAUSE

SYMPTOMS Menopause is not an illness but a natural condition that occurs when the ovaries no longer produce enough oestrogen to stimulate the linings of the uterus and vagina properly. Simply put, menopause is when women no longer menstruate or get pregnant. It generally occurs somewhere between the ages of 40 and 60. One of the most famous signs of menopause is the hot flush, a sudden reddening of the face accompanied by a feeling of intense warmth. Other common symptoms include depressed mood, fluid retention, headache, insomnia, irritability, nervousness, night sweats, painful intercourse, rapid heart beat, susceptibility to bladder problems, thinning of vaginal tissues, vaginal dryness, and weight gain. It should be noted that some women experience few symptoms, while still others encounter none at all.

HOW VITAMIN E CAN HELP The traditional "remedy" for menopause is hormone replacement therapy. This optional treatment uses synthetic hormones to elevate progesterone and oestrogen to their premenopausal levels. Vitamin E is helpful regardless of whether one undergoes or forgoes hormone replacement therapy. A number of researchers believe that the vitamin can improve hot flushes and vaginal dryness, possibly by indirectly affecting hormone levels.

DOSAGES Take up to 800mg of vitamin E daily with meals. Vitamin E oil can be used topically up to twice a day to help treat thinning vaginal tissue and vaginal dryness. In addition, consume daily servings of foods rich in vitamin E, such as avocados, brown rice, dark green leafy vegetables, nuts, oatmeal, seeds, soybeans, and wheatgerm.

CONDITIONS AND DOSES

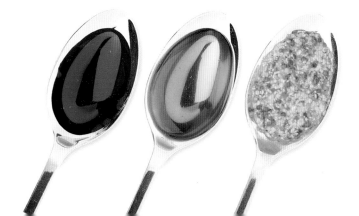

PREMENSTRUAL SYNDROME

SYMPTOMS Premenstrual syndrome, popularly known as PMS, is a predictable pattern of physical and emotional changes that occur in some women just before menstruation. Symptoms range from barely noticeable to extreme and can include abdominal swelling, anxiety, bloating, breast soreness, clumsiness, depressed mood, difficulty concentrating, fatigue, fluid retention, headaches, irritability, lethargy, skin eruptions, sleep disturbances, swollen hands and feet, and weight gain. While it is not known exactly what causes the condition, theories include hormonal, nutritional, and psychological factors.

HOW VITAMIN E CAN HELP Vitamin E is a popular nutritional therapy for PMS. One study found that the vitamin effectively reduced breast soreness, difficulty concentrating, headaches, and irritability. It is not known exactly how the vitamin affects PMS; one theory is that vitamin E has hormone-regulating effects and thus normalizes hormonal levels.

DOSAGES As both a preventative and treatment, take 100–400mg of vitamin E daily with meals. In addition, consume daily servings of foods rich in vitamin E, such as avocados, brown rice, dark green leafy vegetables, nuts, oatmeal, seeds, soybeans, and wheatgerm.

· FERTILITY AID? ·

Infertility is defined as the inability to conceive after a full year of unprotected intercourse. The problem can lie with the male (up to 40 per cent of all cases) or female (up to 60 per cent of all cases). Although medical measures – fertility drugs, in vitro fertilization, donor eggs or sperm – can increase the chance of conceiving, medical intervention is costly, physically invasive, and time consuming. The alternative? Many researchers claim that vitamin E has helped men and women become fertile in the presence of unexplained infertility. Several small studies, including one of the earliest observations of the physiological effects of vitamin E deficiency, have linked vitamin E and reproductive health. In pregnant female animals deficient in vitamin E, foetuses died; in males, the testes became atrophied. Indeed, vitamin E is stored in large amounts in the female and male reproductive organs. But does any of this mean vitamin E can make an infertile person fertile? Unfortunately, no large-scale study has been done on the subject. Right now, the medical establishment views vitamin E's fertility ability as anecdotal.

RHEUMATOID ARTHRITIS

SYMPTOMS Rheumatoid arthritis is an autoimmune disease in which the body's immune system attacks itself. Though the ailment is not well understood, it is believed that an unidentified virus stimulates the body to attack its own joints. Symptoms include pain and swelling in the smaller joints of hands and feet, overall aching and/or stiffness after periods of inactivity, and local fever in affected joints.

HOW VITAMIN E CAN HELP Vitamin E is a helpful companion therapy that can be used in conjunction with other vitamins, herbs, and medications. The vitamin is a powerful antioxidant that protects joints from damage by free radicals, thus increasing joint mobility. Moreover, regular intake of vitamin E has been shown in small studies to lessen rheumatoid arthritis pain.

DOSAGES Take 100–400mg of vitamin E three times daily with meals. In addition, consume daily servings of foods rich in vitamin E, such as avocados, brown rice, dark green leafy vegetables, nuts, oatmeal, seeds, soybeans, and wheatgerm.

· IT'S ALL IN THE DOSAGE ·

An eight-year study in the US found that women who took more than 67mg of vitamin E a day had 36 per cent fewer heart attacks than those who consumed less than 20mg a day.

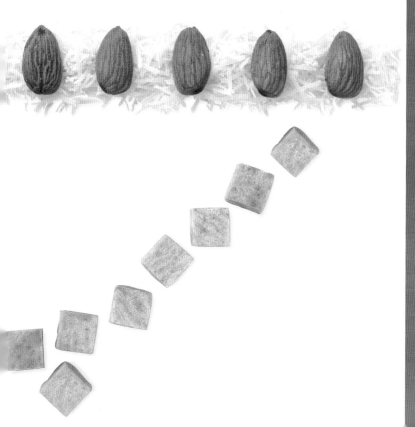

SUNBURN

SYMPTOMS First-degree to second-degree burns caused by the sun's ultraviolet rays leave the affected area red, inflamed, tender, painful, and sometimes blistered. The amount of sun exposure that can cause a burn – also known as ultraviolet skin damage – depends on the amount of protective melanin an individual has in his or her skin, atmospheric conditions, the geographical location, and the time of day.

HOW VITAMIN E CAN HELP Vitamin E cannot prevent sunburn – only sun avoidance, sunblock, and/or protective clothing can do that. What vitamin E can do, according to several new American and German studies, is to help bolster the skin's internal resistance to ultraviolet rays. Studies have found that vitamin E, used topically, can help reduce the incidence of sunburn by 10 to 20 per cent. Vitamin E is a powerful antioxidant that can help prevent free radical damage at a cellular level, thus halting a large amount of ultraviolet damage before it starts.

DOSAGES As a preventative, take 100–400mg of vitamin E orally, and also apply vitamin E cream. In addition, consume daily servings of foods rich in vitamin E, such as avocados, brown rice, dark green leafy vegetables, nuts, oatmeal, seeds, soybeans, and wheatgerm.

· TISSUE REGENERATION ·

While many doctors question vitamin E's effectiveness as a wound-healer, several small studies have found that vitamin E does facilitate healing. After all, vitamin E is necessary for tissue generation, so it makes sense that it can help mend wounds. To try it yourself, wait a day or two for the cut to close, then gently rub vitamin E oil onto the affected area. Repeat up to twice a day. Puncture capsules of the vitamin and squeeze out the contents for application; or head to the health food store, where you can purchase a small bottle of vitamin E oil.

ALTERNATIVE HEALTH STRATEGIES

Herbs, vitamins, and minerals all contribute to good health. However, creating a sense of general well-being involves more than simply taking supplements. Health has to do with a quality of life that can often be aggravated by causes of harmful stress. Listed below are some additional ways to help keep yourself well.

IMPROVE YOUR EATING HABITS

Here are the five main eating strategies people follow; consider finding the healthiest one that works with your lifestyle.

- Omnivore
- Semi-vegetarian
- Macrobiotic
- Vegan
- Vegetarian

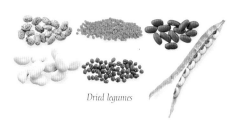

Dried legumes

GET MORE EXERCISE

Whether it's walking or weightlifting, any type of exercise can help you feel better. Try any of these types:

- Stretching
- Aerobics
- Resistance training

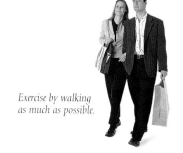

Exercise by walking as much as possible.

SIMPLE WAYS TO EASE STRESS

In addition to exercise and healthy eating, here are some more techniques – old and new – for easing stress and increasing relaxation.

- Get enough sleep
- Take time to relax
- Give up junk food
- Adopt a pet
- Surround yourself with supportive people
- Limit your exposure to chemicals
- Enjoy yourself

· ONE-MINUTE STRESS REDUCER ·

Deep breathing can be done anywhere and anytime you need to calm and centre yourself:

1 Inhale deeply through your nose.
2 Hold your breath for up to three seconds, then exhale your breath through your mouth.
3 Continue as needed.

Deep breathing draws a person's attention away from a given stress and refocuses it on his or her breathing. This type of breathing is not only comforting (thanks to its rhythmic quality), but also has been shown to lower rapid pulse and shallow respiration – two temporary symptoms of stress.

GET MOVING

Ask medical experts to name one stay-young strategy and there's a good chance that "exercise" will be the answer. And with good reason. Exercise, whether a gentle walk around the block or a full-tilt weight lifting session, strengthens the heart, lowers the body's resting heart rate, builds muscles, boosts circulation to the body and the brain, revs up the metabolism and burns calories. All of which can keep a person looking and feeling his or her best. For it to be effective, exercise several times a week. Aim for at least three sessions. For optimum health, try a combination of aerobic exercise and strength training. And don't forget to stretch before and after each workout!

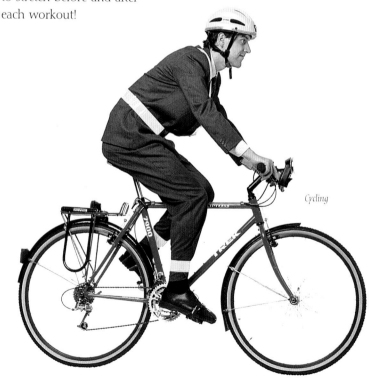

Cycling

STRETCHING

WHAT IT IS Any movement that stretches muscles. Examples include bending at the waist and touching the toes, sitting with legs outstretched in front of you, and rolling your neck. Stretch for eight to 12 minutes before every workout and again after you exercise.

WHY IT'S IMPORTANT Muscles act like springs. If a muscle is short and tight, it loses the ability to absorb shock. The less shock a muscle can absorb, the more strain there is on the joints. Thus, stretching maintains flexibility, which in turn prevents injuries. Because we often lose our regular range of motion with age, stretching is especially important for older adults to prevent sprains, strains and falls.

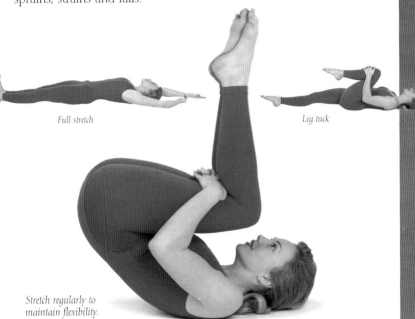

Full stretch

Leg tuck

Stretch regularly to maintain flexibility.

AEROBICS

WHAT IT IS Any activity that uses large muscle groups, is maintained continuously for 15 minutes or more, and is rhythmic in nature. Examples include aerobic dance, jogging, skating and walking. Ideally, you should aim for three to six aerobic workouts per week.

WHY IT'S IMPORTANT Aerobic exercise trains the heart, lungs, and cardiovascular system to process and deliver oxygen more quickly and efficiently to every part of the body. As the heart muscle becomes stronger and more efficient, a larger amount of blood can be pumped with each stroke. Fewer strokes are then required to rapidly transport oxygen to all parts of the body.

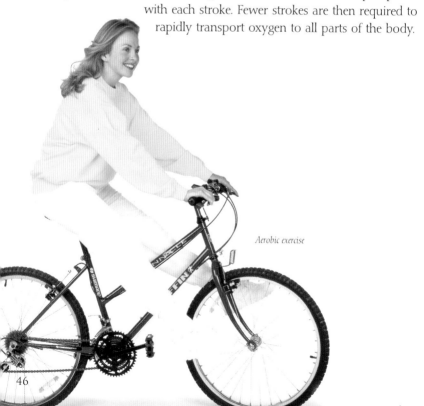

Aerobic exercise

RESISTANCE TRAINING

WHAT IT IS Any activity that improves the condition of your muscles by making repeated movements against a force. Examples include lifting large or small weights, sit-ups, stair-stepping, and isometrics.

WHY IT'S IMPORTANT Resistance training makes it easier to move heavy loads, whether they require carrying, pushing, pulling, or lifting, as well as participating in sports that require strength. The exercises are of various kinds. Some require changing the length of the muscle while maintaining the level of tension, others involve using special equipment to vary the tension in the muscles, and some entail contracting a muscle while maintaining its length.

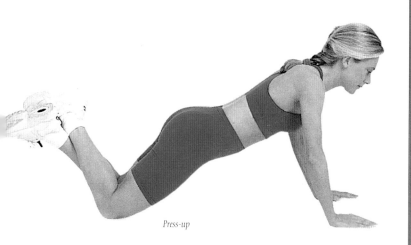

Press-up

EATING SMART

A balanced diet is the foundation of good health. For proof, just read the numerous medical studies that link healthy eating with disease prevention and disease reversal. These same studies connect high fat intake, high sodium consumption, and diets with too much protein to numerous illnesses, including cancer, cardiovascular diseases, diverticular diseases, hypertension, and heart disease. But what exactly is a balanced diet? Generally speaking, it is a diet comprised of carbohydrates, dietary fibre, fat, protein, water, 13 vitamins and 20 minerals. More specifically, it is a diet built around a wide variety of fruits, legumes, whole grains, and vegetables. Alcohol, animal protein, high-fat foods, high-sodium foods, highly-sugared foods, fizzy drinks, and processed foods are consumed sparingly.

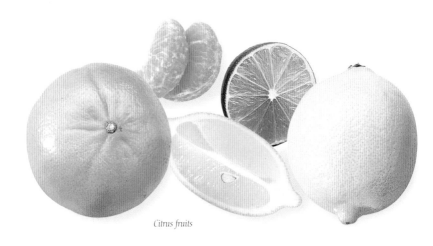

Citrus fruits

OMNIVOROUS

ON THE MENU Plant-based foods, dairy products, eggs, fish, seafood, red meats, organ meats, poultry.

FOODS THAT ARE AVOIDED None. Everything is fair game.

Egg

HOW HEALTHY IS IT? It depends. Someone who eats eggs, poultry, or meat every day, chooses refined snacks over whole foods, and gets only one or two daily servings of fruits and vegetables will not be as healthy as a person who limits meat (the general dietary term for any "flesh foods", including poultry and fish) to two or three times a week, chooses water over soft drinks, and gets the recommended five or more daily servings of fruits and vegetables. Complaints about traditional omnivorous diets revolve around the diet's high levels of cholesterol and saturated fat (found in animal-based foods), which increase the risk of cancer, diabetes, heart disease, and obesity. However, an omnivorous diet can be healthful one provided thoughtful choices are made. To keep cholesterol and saturated fat to a minimum and nutrients to a maximum, eat five or more daily servings of fruits and vegetables, choose whole grains over refined grains, enjoy daily legume or soyfood protein sources, and limit the use of animal foods.

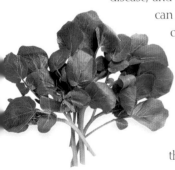

Watercress

MACROBIOTIC

ON THE MENU Plant-based foods, fish, very limited amounts of salt.

FOODS THAT ARE AVOIDED Dairy products, eggs, foods with artificial ingredients, hot spices, mass-produced foods, organ meats, peppers, potatoes, poultry, red meats, shellfish, warm drinks, and refined foods.

HOW HEALTHY IS IT? Macrobiotics is based on a system created in the early 1900s by Japanese philosopher George Ohsawa. The diet consists of 50 per cent whole grains, 20-30 per cent vegetables, and 5-10 per cent beans, sea vegetables, and soy foods. The remainder of the diet is composed of white-meat fish, fruits, and nuts. The diet's low amounts of saturated fat, absence of processed foods, and emphasis on high-fibre foods such as whole grains and vegetables, may promote cardiovascular health. Because soy and sea vegetables contain cancer-fighting compounds, a macrobiotic diet is often recommended to help treat cancer. However, critics worry that the diet's limited variety of food can leave followers lacking in certain vitamins and important cancer-fighting phytonutrients.

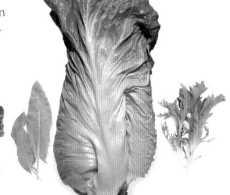

Leafy green vegetables

SEMI-VEGETARIAN

ON THE MENU Plant-based foods, dairy products, eggs, fish, seafood.

FOODS THAT ARE AVOIDED Red meats, organ meats, poultry.

HOW HEALTHY IS IT? Like an omnivorous diet, a semi-vegetarian diet is as healthy as a person makes it. Individuals who eat high-fat and highly processed foods fail to get the recommended daily number of vegetables and fruits, and eschew whole grains for processed grains will not enjoy optimum health. That said, individuals who are conscientious about eating a balanced, varied diet, and who limit fish and seafood intake to two or three times per week, can expect a lower risk of heart disease. Since many oily fish contain omega-3 fatty acids, eating them in moderation has been found to help lower blood cholesterol. Be aware, however, that oily saltwater fish such as shark, swordfish and tuna have been found to carry mercury in their tissues; many health authorities recommend eating these varieties no more than once or twice a week. Also, due to overfishing, many fish species are now threatened, including bluefin tuna, Pacific perch, Chilean sea bass, Chinook salmon, and swordfish.

Shellfish

VEGAN

ON THE MENU Plant-based foods.

FOODS THAT ARE AVOIDED Dairy, eggs, fish, seafood, red meats, organ meats, poultry. Also avoided are foods made by animals or processed with animal parts, such as gelatin, honey, marshmallows made with animal gelatin, white sugar processed with bone char.

HOW HEALTHY IS IT? A vegan (pronounced VEE-gun) diet can be extremely healthful. Like the vegetarian diet, a vegan diet has been shown by numerous studies to lower blood pressure and prevent heart disease. In addition, the high fibre intake cuts the risk of diverticular disease and colon cancer. Yet because vegans do not eat dairy products or eggs, they must be more conscientious than vegetarians about eating plant foods with vitamin B12 and vitamin D or taking supplements of these nutrients.

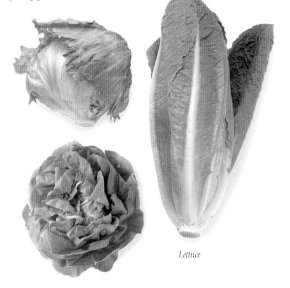

Lettuce

VEGETARIAN

ON THE MENU Plant-based foods, dairy, eggs.

FOODS THAT ARE AVOIDED Fish, gelatin, seafood, red meats, organ meats, poultry.

HOW HEALTHY IS IT? A vegetarian diet can be very healthy when done right. Fortunately, this isn't hard. Dietary science has debunked theories of "protein combining" popular in the 1960s and 1970s, leaving today's vegetarians to worry only about eating a wide variety of whole foods including beans, fruits, grains, low-fat dairy products, nuts, soy foods, and vegetables. A varied daily diet insures enough protein, calcium, and other nutrients for vegetarians of all ages, including children, pregnant individuals, and the elderly. A well-chosen vegetarian eating plan has been shown by numerous studies to lower blood pressure, decrease the risk of breast cancer, and prevent heart disease. In addition, the diet's high fibre levels cut the risk of diverticular disease and colon cancer.

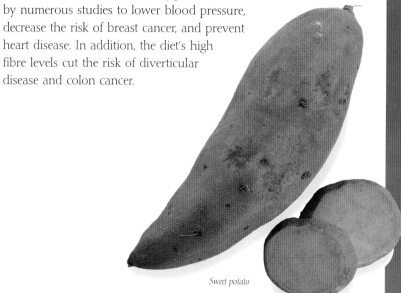

Sweet potato

NUTRIENT KNOW-HOW

Vitamins and minerals are known collectively as nutrients. Name a body function such as carbohydrate metabolism, nerve cell replication, or wound healing and you'll find one or more of these nutrients at work. The best place to look for vitamins and minerals? In the food you eat every day. Indeed, if you eat a well-balanced diet

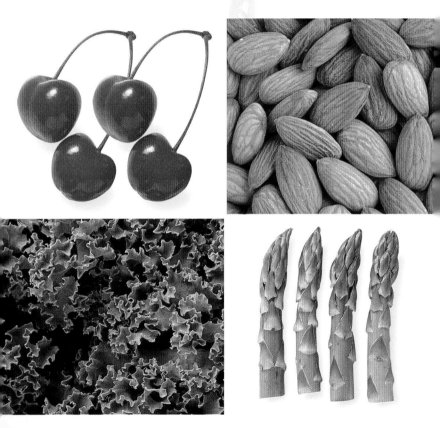

there is a good chance you'll get all the nutrients your body needs. But if you are ill, pregnant, eat an inadequate diet, drink more than two alcoholic or caffeinated drinks per day, are under stress, are taking certain medications, or have difficulty absorbing certain nutrients, you may need to supplement your diet with one or more vitamins or minerals. Supplements generally come in tablet and capsule form, although some health food stores also carry liquid supplements. Whichever form you choose, doses are measured by weight in milligrams (mg); in micrograms (mcg); or in the universal standard known as international units (IU).

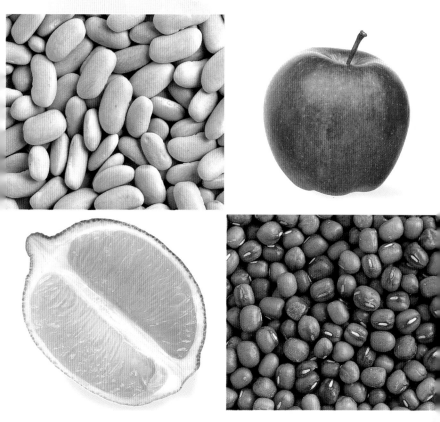

VITAMIN A
(beta carotene, retinol)

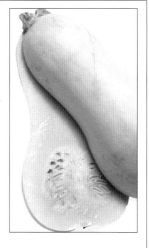

What It Does Vitamin A is found in two forms: performed vitamin A, known as retinol, and provitamin A, called beta carotene. Retinol is found only in foods of animal origin. Beta carotene, a carotenoid, is a pigment found in plants. Beta carotene has a slight nutritional edge, boasting antioxidant properties and the ability to help lower harmful cholesterol levels. Regardless of the form, vitamin A is essential for good vision, promotes healthy skin, hair, and mucous membranes, stimulates wound healing, and is necessary for the proper development of bones and teeth.

EU Recommended Daily Allowance 800µg.
Food Sources: Orange and yellow fruits and vegetables, dark green leafy vegetables, whole milk, cream, butter, organ meats.

Toxic Dosage When taken excessively vitamin A can cause abdominal pain, amenorrhoea, dry skin, enlarged liver or spleen, hair loss, headaches, itching, joint pain, nausea, vision problems, vomiting.

Enemies Antibiotics, cholesterol-lowering drugs, heavy laxative use.

Deficiency Symptoms Because vitamin A is fat-soluble, it is stored in the body's fat for a long time, making deficiency uncommon. However, deficiency symptoms include dryness of the conjunctiva and cornea, frequent colds, insomnia, night blindness, reproductive difficulties, and respiratory infections.

VITAMIN B₁
(thiamine)

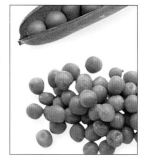

What It Does Maintains normal nervous system functioning, helps metabolize carbohydrates, proteins, and fats; assists in blood formation and circulation; optimizes cognitive activity and brain function; regulates the body's appetite; protects the body from the degenerative effects of alcohol consumption, environmental pollution, and smoking.

Minimum Recommended Daily Allowance 1.4mg.

Food Sources Brewer's yeast, broccoli, brown rice, egg yolks, fish, legumes, peanuts, peas, pork, prunes, oatmeal, raisins, rice bran, soybeans, wheatgerm, whole grains.

Toxic Dosage There is no know toxicity level for vitamin B1.
Enemies: Antibiotics, a diet high in simple carbohydrates, heavy physical exertion, oral contraceptives.

Deficiency Symptoms Appetite loss, confusion, fatigue, heart arrhythmia, nausea, mood swings. Severe deficiency can lead to beriberi, a crippling disease characterized by convulsions, diarrhoea, edema, gastrointestinal problems, heart failure, mental confusion, nerve damage, paralysis, and severe weight loss.

VITAMIN B₂
(riboflavin, vitamin G)

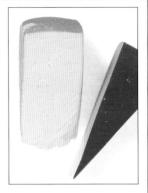

What It Does Helps metabolize carbohydrates, fats, and proteins; allows skin, nail, and hair tissues to utilize oxygen; aids in red blood cell formation and antibody production; promotes cell respiration; maintains proper nerve function, eyes, and adrenal glands.
Minimum Recommended Daily Allowance 1.6mg.
Food Sources Cheese, egg yolks, fish, legumes, milk, poultry, spinach, whole grains, yoghurt.
Toxic Dosage There is no known toxicity level for this vitamin, although nervousness and rapid heartbeat have been reported with daily dosages of 10mg.
Enemies Alcohol, oral contraceptives, strenuous exercise.
Deficiency Symptoms Cracks at the corners of the mouth, dermatitis, dizziness, hair loss, insomnia, itchy or burning eyes, light sensitivity, mouth sores, impaired thinking, inflammation of the tongue, rashes.

VITAMIN B₅
(pantothenic acid)

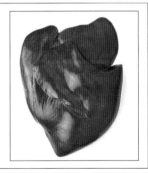

What It Does Helps produce adrenal hormones, antibodies, and various neurotransmitters; reduces skin inflammation; speeds healing of wounds; helps convert food to energy.
Minimum Recommended Daily Allowance 6mg.
Food Sources Beef, eggs, beans, brown rice, corn, lentils, mushrooms, nuts, peas, pork, saltwater fish, sweet potatoes.
Toxic Dosages There is no known toxicity level for this vitamin; however, doses above 10mg can cause diarrhoea in some individuals.
Deficiency Symptoms Vitamin B5 deficiency is extremely rare and is likely to occur only with starvation.

VITAMIN B₆
(pyridoxine)

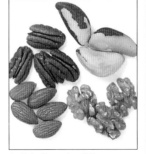

What It Does Involved in more bodily functions than nearly any other nutrient. It helps the body metabolize carbohydrates, fats and proteins; supports immune function; helps build red blood cells; assists in transmission of nerve impulses; maintains the body's sodium and potassium balance; helps synthesize RNA and DNA.
Minimum Recommended Daily Allowance 2mg.
Food Sources Avocados, bananas, beans, blackstrap molasses, brown rice, carrots, corn, fish, nuts, sunflower seeds.
Toxic Dosage Levels of over 500mg can cause numbness in the hands and feet.
Deficiency Symptoms Vitamin B6 deficiency is rare. Symptoms include depression, fatigue, flaky skin, headaches, insomnia, irritability, muscle weakness, nausea.

VITAMIN B₁₂
(cobalamin)

What It Does Regulates formation of red blood cells, helps the body utilize iron; converts carbohydrates, fats, and proteins into energy; aids in cellular formation and cellular longevity; prevents nerve damage; maintains fertility; promotes normal growth.
Minimum Recommended Daily Allowance 1μg.
Food Sources Brewer's yeast, dairy products, eggs, organ meats, seafood, sea vegetables.
Toxic Dosage There is no known toxicity level for vitamin B12.
Enemies Anti-coagulant drugs, anti-gout medication, potassium supplements.
Deficiency Symptoms While deficiency is rare, individuals who do not eat animal products are at risk unless they fortify their diets with plant-sources such as brewer's yeast and sea vegetables. Symptoms include back pain, body odour, constipation, dizziness, fatigue, moodiness, numbness and tingling in the arms and legs, ringing in the ears, muscle weakness, tongue inflammation, weight loss. Severe deficiency can lead to pernicious anaemia, characterized by abdominal pain, stiffness in the arms and legs, a tendency to bleed, yellowish cast to the skin, permanent nerve damage, death.

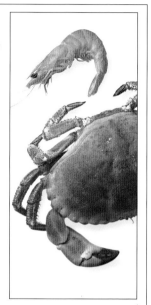

VITAMIN C
(ascorbic acid)

What It Does Protects against pollution and infection, enhances immunity; aids in growth and repair of both bone and tissue by helping the body produce collagen; maintains adrenal gland function; helps the body absorb iron; aids in production of anti-stress hormones; reduces cholesterol levels; lowers high blood pressure; prevents artherosclerosis.
Minimum Recommended Daily Allowance 60mg.
Food Sources Berries, cantaloupe, citrus fruits, broccoli, leafy greens, mangoes, papayas, peppers, persimmons, pineapple, tomatoes.
Toxic Dosage Doses larger than 10,000mg can cause diarrhoea, stomach irritation, or increased kidney stone formation.
Enemies Alcohol, analgesics, antidepressants, anticoagulants, oral contraceptives, smoking, steroids.
Deficiency Symptoms Bleeding gums, easy bruising, fatigue, reduced resistance to colds and other infections, slow healing of wounds, weight loss. Severe deficiency can lead to scurvy, a sometimes-fatal disease characterized by aching bones, muscle weakness, and swollen and bleeding gums.

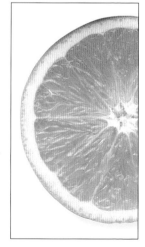

VITAMIN D
(calciferol, ergosterol)

What It Does Helps the body utilize calcium and phosphorus; promotes normal development of bones and teeth; assists in thyroid function; maintains normal blood clotting; helps regulate heartbeat, nerve function, and muscle contraction.
Minimum Recommended Daily Allowance 5µg
Food Sources Dandelion greens, dairy products, eggs, fatty saltwater fish, parsley, sweet potatoes, vegetable oils.
Toxic Dosage Daily doses higher than 20µg can lead to raised blood calcium levels and calcium deposits of the heart, liver, and kidney.
Enemies Antacids, cholesterol-lowering drugs, cortisone drugs.
Deficiency Symptoms The body naturally manufactures about 200 IU of vitamin D when exposed to ten minutes of ultraviolet light, making deficiency rare. Symptoms include bone weakening, diarrhoea, insomnia, muscle twitches, vision disturbances. Severe deficiency can lead to rickets, a disease that results in bone defects such as bowlegs and knock-knees.

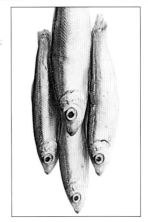

VITAMIN E
(tocopherol)

What It Does Prevents unstable molecules known as free radicals from damaging cells and tissue; accelerates wound healing; protects lung tissue from inhaled pollutants; aids in functioning of the immune system; endocrine system, and sex glands; improves circulation; promotes normal blood clotting.
Minimum Recommended Daily Allowance 10mg
Food Sources Avocados, dark green leafy vegetables, eggs, legumes, nuts, organ meats, seafood, seeds, soybeans.
Toxic Dosage Although there is no established toxicity level of vitamin E, the vitamin has blood-thinning properties; individuals who are taking anticoagulant medications or have clotting deficiencies should avoid vitamin E at doses higher than 800mg.
Enemies High temperatures and overcooking reduce vitamin E levels in food.
Deficiency Symptoms Vitamin E deficiency is rare. Deficiency symptoms include fluid retention, infertility, miscarriage, muscle degeneration.

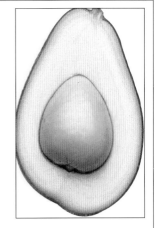

CALCIUM

What It Does Necessary for the growth and maintenance of bones, teeth, and healthy gums; maintains normal blood pressure normal; may reduce risk of heart disease; enables muscles, including the heart, to contract; is essential for normal blood clotting; needed for proper nerve impulse transmission; maintains connective tissue; helps prevent rickets and osteoporosis.
Minimum Recommended Daily Allowance 800mg.
Food Sources Asparagus, cruciferous vegetables, dairy products, dark leafy vegetables, figs, legumes, nuts, oats, prunes, salmon with bones, sardines with bones, seeds, soybeans, tofu.
Toxic Dosage Daily intake of 2,000mg or more can lead to constipation, calcium deposits in the soft tissue, urinary tract infections, and possible interference with the body's absorption of zinc.
Enemies Alcohol, caffeine, excessive sugar intake, high-protein diet, high sodium intake, inadequate levels of vitamin D, soft drinks containing phosphorous.
Deficiency Symptoms Aching joints, brittle nails, eczema, elevated blood cholesterol, heart palpitations, hypertension, insomnia, muscle cramps, nervousness, pallor, tooth decay.

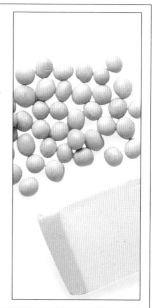

IRON

What It Does Aids in the production of haemoglobin (the protein in red blood cells that transports oxygen from the lungs to the body's tissue) and myoglobin (a protein that provides extra fuel to muscles during exertion); helps maintain healthy immune system; is important for growth.
Minimum Recommended Daily Allowance 14mg.
Food Sources Beef, blackstrap molasses, brewer's yeast, dark green vegetables, dried fruit, legumes, nuts, organ meats, sea vegetables, seeds, soybeans, whole grains.
Toxic Dosage Iron should not be taken in excess of 35mg daily without a doctor's recommendation. In high doses, iron can cause diarrhoea, dizziness, fatigue, headaches, stomach-aches, weakened pulse. Excess iron inhibits the absorption of phosphorus and vitamin E, interferes with immune function, and has been associated with cancer, cirrhosis, heart disease.
Enemies Antacids, caffeine, tetracycline, iron absorption, excessive menstrual bleeding, long-term illness, an ulcer.
Deficiency Symptoms Anaemia, brittle hair, difficulty swallowing, dizziness, fatigue, hair loss, irritability, nervousness, pallor, ridges on the nails, sensitivity to cold, slowed mental reactions.

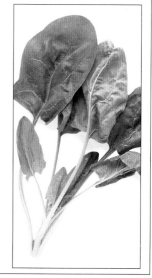

MAGNESIUM

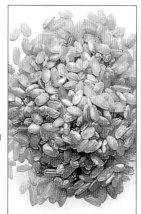

What It Does Plays a role in formation of bone; protects arterial linings from stress caused by sudden blood pressure; helps body metabolize carbohydrates and minerals; assists in building proteins; helps maintain healthy bones and teeth; reduces the risk of developing osteoporosis.
Minimum Recommended Daily Allowance 300mg.
Food Sources Apples, apricots, avocados, bananas, blackstrap molasses, brewer's yeast. brown rice, cantaloupe, dairy products, figs, garlic, green leafy vegetables, legumes, nuts.
Toxic Dosage Daily doses over 3,000mg can lead to diarrhoea, fatigue, muscle weakness, and in extreme cases, severely depressed heart rate and blood pressure, shallow breathing, loss of reflexes and coma.
Enemies Alcohol, diuretics, high-fat intake, high-protein diet.
Deficiency Symptoms Though deficiency is rare, symptoms include disorientation, heart palpitations, listlessness, muscle weakness.

POTASSIUM

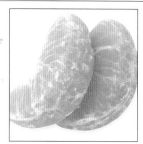

What It Does Maintains a healthy nervous system and regular heart rhythm; helps prevent stroke; aids in proper muscle contractions; controls the body's water balance; assists chemical reactions within cells; aids in the transmission of electrochemical impulses; maintains stable blood pressure; required for protein synthesis, carbohydrate metabolism, and insulin secretion by the pancreas.
No EU Recommended Daily Allowance
Food Sources Apricots, avocados, bananas, blackstrap molasses, brewer's yeast, brown rice, citrus fruits, dairy.
Toxic Dosage Should not be taken in excess of 18 grams.
Enemies Diarrhoea, diuretics, caffeine use, heavy perspiration, kidney disorders, tobacco use.
Deficiency Symptoms Chills, dry skin, constipation, depression, diminished reflexes, edema, headaches, insatiable thirst, fluctuations in heartbeat, nervousness, respiratory distress.

ZINC

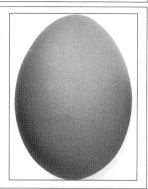

What It Does Contributes to a wide range of bodily processes. Aids in cell respiration; assists in bone development; helps energy metabolism, promotes wound healing; regulates heart rate and blood pressure; helps liver remove toxic substances, such as alcohol, from the body.
Minimum Recommended Daily Allowance 15mg
Food Sources Brewer's yeast, cheese, egg yolks, lamb, legumes, mushrooms, nuts, organ meats, sea food, sea vegetables, seeds.
Toxic Dosage Do not take more than 50mg zinc daily. In doses higher than this zinc can depress the immune system.
Deficiency Symptoms Appetite loss, dermatitis, fatigue, impaired wound healing, loss of taste, white streaks on the nails.

INDEX

ACKNOWLEDGEMENTS

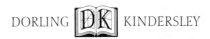

DORLING KINDERSLEY

LONDON, NEW YORK, SYDNEY, DEHLI, PARIS,
MUNICH, and JOHANNESBURG

Stephanie Pedersen is an American writer and editor who specializes in the
area of health. Her articles have appeared in numerous publications and she
has also co-written several books published by St. Martin's Press.

The publisher would like to thank Norma McGough BSc Hons FRD for
acting as UK consultant on the series.

Editorial Director: LaVonne Carlson
Editors: Nancy Burke, Barbara Minton, Connie Robinson
Designer: Carol Wells
Cover Designer: Gus Yoo

Picture Credits: Steve Gorton, David Murray, Dave King, Martin Norris,
Philip Gatward, Andy Crawford, Philip Dowell, Clive Streeter, Peter Chadwick,
Tim Ridley, Andrew Whittack, Martin Cameron

Copyright © 2001 Dorling Kindersley Limited

First published in Great Britain in 2001 by
Dorling Kindersley Limited
9 Henrietta Street, London, WC2E 8PS

2 4 6 8 10 9 7 5 3 1

All rights reserved. No part of this book may be reproduced, stored in a retrieval system, or
transmitted in any form or by any means, electronic, mechanical, photocopying, recording
or otherwise, without the prior written permission of the copyright owners.

A CIP catalogue record for this book is available from the British Library

ISBN 0 7513 31023

Reproduction by Dai Nippon Printing Co., (HK Ltd.)
Printed and bound in China by L.Rex Printing Co., Ltd.

see our complete catalogue at
www.dk.com